Adhering to Your Medication

Dr. Talya Miron-Shatz and the Buddy&Soul team

Taking your medication is vital, especially when it comes to optimizing your long-term health. And yet, if you're taking this course, you know how hard it is to take your medication in a timely and efficient manner. And to do it all the time! This course offers you a fresh new look into adhering to your medication by exploring the cognitive, emotional, and behavioral elements that may be preventing you from improving your medication adherence, and your health outcomes.

You may be feeling pretty good, as far as suffering from an illness goes.

Maybe you and your doctor have just decided together on the best treatment plan for you and you're quite optimistic about what needs to be done.

Well, what happens now?

Unfortunately, if you're like most patients, you'll likely find that even **all the optimism in the world won't necessarily translate into a perfect adherence score on your part**.

In simplified terms, adherence is how well you follow your treatment plan. This can refer to taking medicine, making lifestyle and dietary changes, or whatever helps keep your condition under control.

I know from my own first-hand experience that just getting involved in a new project or having to travel can throw me off and make me forget to take my own meds. And that's me – a smart, dedicated lady, and very mindful of my health!

For a combination of reasons, no matter how good patients feel about their physician, their treatment, or the idea of lifestyle changes, most of them somehow don't find themselves following through as well as they should or could.

This course is intended to help you bridge that gap.

We'll identify what holds you back from optimal adherence, explore research-based strategies to help you up your game, and empower you to assume greater responsibility for your health decisions.

We believe what we've put together here can really make a difference.

So, whether you are a member of the "long-term chronic illness club" or your stint with medication is short-term, this course can help you improve your adherence and, most importantly, your health.

There are three goals that we had in mind while creating this book. We want you to:

1. Delve a little deeper into what may be holding you back from optimal adherence.
2. Learn practical tools to help ensure you take your meds as needed.
3. Assume responsibility for how you handle adherence to medication.

If your adherence is anything short of perfect, this course is for you!

YOUR JOURNEY TO ADHERING TO YOUR MEDICATION

HOW TO USE THIS BOOK TO ADHERE TO YOUR MEDICATION

In this book you'll find ten great strategies for achieving the goals we listed above. You'll also find inspiring content and exercises you can engage with to help you practice emotionally managing your illness. You will get the most out of this book by going through the strategies and associated exercises one by one. Of course, you can also simply read it the whole way through. But we recommend using this book by going through it in order, watching the TED talks, and doing the exercises. We have found the best way to do the exercises is by dedicating a notebook as your course journal. If you're reading this book on a PC, feel free to create a text file and use that as your course journal. Or you could simply use a good ol' pen and paper to do the exercises. Either way, we recommend keeping some method of writing handy while you go through the exercises in this book to optimize what you get out of it.

To maximize your experience with the Buddy and Soul book, share your thoughts and insights with us on social media! Post pictures relating to your progress on Instagram and Twitter, tagging @Buddy_N_Soul, and Facebook @Buddy&Soul.   By sharing with us on social media, not only can you help others with their personal journeys, you can read about those facing similar challenges.

Direct message us YOUR story @Buddy_N_Soul on Instagram and be anonymously featured for a chance to **win a Buddy&Soul three month free membership**.

If you really want to go all the way, visit our website, BuddynSoul.com, and explore all that we have to offer beyond 'Emotionally Managing your Illness'. In fact, we have two other books in the Medical Series that we think you might benefit from: Emotionally Manage Your Illness and Manage Your Medical Condition

WHY I CREATED BUDDY&SOUL AND WHY I CREATED THIS BOOK

I'm Dr. Talya Miron-Shatz, CEO of Buddy&Soul, where Emotionally Managing Your Illness and many more e-courses and books come from. I have a PhD in psychology and was very fortunate to do my post-doc at Princeton University with Nobel Laureate Daniel Kahneman. I've also taught at the Wharton Business School, University of Pennsylvania. Now I'm a professor at the Ono Academic College, and a visiting researcher at Cambridge University. I used to study happiness, and for a long time now, I've been studying medical decision making and helping

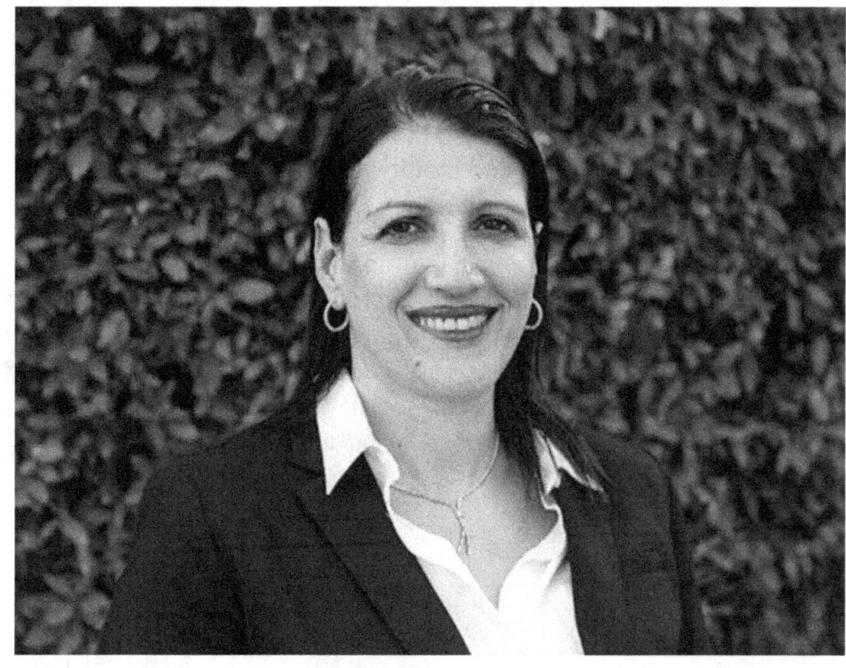

organizations support people on their way to joy and health. One thing that struck me as unfair was that we were expecting people to change their life for good but weren't giving them the tools to do so. People deserve all the help they can get when breaking out of old patterns and moving their lives forward.

This is what Buddy&Soul does.

We support you in many ways by providing science-based actionable ways to sustain your body and mind. We help you sleep better, spark a change in your eating habits, and manage stress. We teach you how to create new habits and how to engage your willpower. We help you grow, claim your self-esteem, cultivate authenticity, reframe your life story, achieve your goals and so much more including Adhering To Your Medication.

Everything you need to change your life for good.

I want to hear from YOU! Please feel free to send me an email with your thoughts, suggestions, and feedback regarding this book to talya@buddynsoul.com. I would love to hear what you think about this book and how it helped you with adhering to your medication. Your feedback is extremely valuable and will allow us to help more individuals, like yourself, to obtain the necessary tools and support needed to change their lives for good.

How I realized I needed help with my adherence

Sometimes we can fake it for months or even years, and sometimes, very early on, we get a wake-up call that reminds us that we need help in order to properly take our meds. How did you realize that your adherence needed a boost, and that it was time for some help?

Take some time brainstorming in your journal about your experience with medication, and then share your story with the Buddy and Soul community! Tag us on Instagram and Twitter @Buddy_N_Soul, using the **#BuddynSoulMedSupport**. You can also direct message us YOUR story @Buddy_N_Soul on Instagram and be anonymously featured for a chance to **win a Buddy&Soul three month free membership**. By sharing with us on social media, not only can you help others with their personal journeys, you can read about those facing similar challenges.

9 Benefits of adhering to your medication

Of course, when you take your meds properly, you're doing your medical condition a favor. But there are many side benefits of proper adherence that have little to do with the direct workings of your medication. Read on to see how medication adherence can benefit you in other ways too.

1. Knowing that you are doing your part in keeping your medical condition under control builds self-confidence.
2. You are secure in the knowledge that [insert medical mishap here- e.g. a recent flare-up, a sudden change in your condition, etc.] didn't occur as a result of your not taking your meds properly.
3. Only by taking your medicine properly can you discern whether or not it's working for you.
4. The initial kick-in period is shortest when you expose your body to the treatment at the proper intervals and dosages.
5. Getting your money's worth, if you are paying out of pocket.
6. A sense of relief at your upcoming doctor's appointment – you have nothing to be embarrassed

Add your own:

7. ____

8. ____

9. ____

Will learning about adherence actually help me take my meds?

I didn't need to learn about the digestive tract to learn how to chew, or the ins and outs of a car before I learned to drive. Adherence is something you learn from life experience. It doesn't need to be philosophized about!

For:

1. I can learn from others' mistakes, prepare myself, and take precautions not to fall into known traps. Knowledge is power.
2. Better the devil you know than the devil you don't.

Add your own argument:

3. ____

Against:

1. There is a long way from the head to the heart. I can know something intellectually, but I won't necessarily change my day-to-day decisions unless I *feel* the impacts of my poor compliance.
2. I know everything I possibly can about adherence and still, I don't adhere. I am a walking contradiction, just like so many other patients out there. So much for knowledge…

Add your own argument:

3. ____

Medicine, at its best, only works insofar as it's actually taken. In a staple research paper on adherence published in 1999, researchers from University College London found that one of the things that affect how scrupulously patients take their medication is how much they believe in it.

Does this sound a little quirky? Well, think of it this way: If you were handed a magical elixir and told that taking it eleven times a day while standing on one foot and dressed like a giant hot dog would literally make you 10 years younger, would you even bother renting the costume? Chances are that not so much. If you don't believe a medicine can help you, for whatever reason, you're less likely to adhere to it.

And what if you find that you don't actually believe in the necessity or efficacy of your meds? What if you fear its side-effects are worse than the benefits it offers? Does that mean you're doomed to a lifetime of sub-par medical care and disappointed looks from your doctor?

Thankfully, not at all. Once we address our belief about our medication, we can move forward with strengthening and maintaining it.

EXERCISE

Step 1: **Take this survey** (based on the Belief in Medicines Questionnaire) **to gauge your belief in your medication.** Read each of the following statements and rate the level at which you agree on a scale of 1 to 5, with 1 being strongly disagree and 5 being strongly agree.

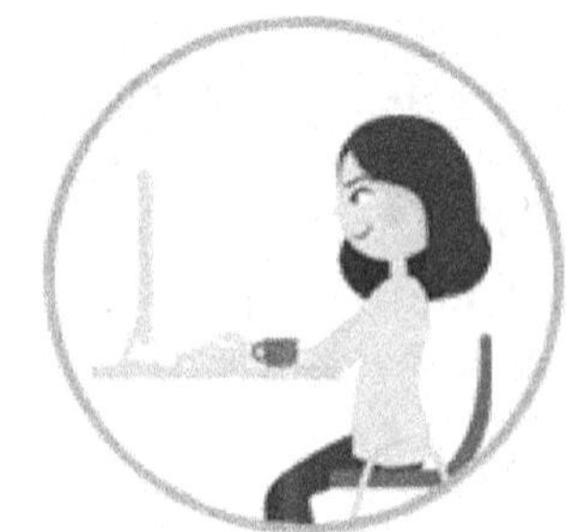

1) My health at present depends on my medicines.

2) Having to take medication worries me.

3) My life would be impossible without my medication.

4) Without my medication I would be very ill.

5) I sometimes worry about the long term effects of my medication.

6) My medication is mystery to me.

7) My health in the future will depend on my medication.

8) My medication disrupts my life.

9) I sometimes worry about becoming too dependent on my medication.

10) My medication protects me from becoming worse.

11) Doctors use too many medicines.

12) People who take medicines should stop their treatment for a while every now and again.

13) Most medicines are addictive.

14) Natural remedies are safer than medicines.

15) Medicines do more harm than good.

16) All medicines are poisons.

17) Doctors place too much trust in medicines.

18) If doctors had more time with patients they would prescribe fewer medicines.

Question #:	What it's worth:				
	1	2	3	4	5
1.	1	2	3	4	5
2. (r)	5	4	3	2	1
3.	1	2	3	4	5
4.	1	2	3	4	5
5. (r)	5	4	3	2	1
6. (r)	5	4	3	2	1
7.	1	2	3	4	5
8. (r)	5	4	3	2	1
9. (r)	5	4	3	2	1
10	1	2	3	4	5
11 (r)	5	4	3	2	1
12 (r)	5	4	3	2	1
13 (r)	5	4	3	2	1
14 (r)	5	4	3	2	1
15 (r)	5	4	3	2	1
16 (r)	5	4	3	2	1
17 (r)	5	4	3	2	1
18(r)	5	4	3	2	1

Rating = all scores combined (including the ones that have been reversed)

Scoring key:

18-42 Low: Your level of faith in your meds and how they're prescribed, as well as in meds in general is low. It might be a good idea to have an open discussion about this with your doc, as lack of faith may reduce adherence to medication.

43–66 Medium: You are on the fence about your meds, and meds in general. It's not that you're against them, but you're also not super-pro. This course can be very helpful for you.

MAX: 67-90 High: Your level of faith in your medication, as well as in doctors' prescribing habits, and in meds in general, is high. This can lead to high adherence. Bravo! This course will help you work with what you've already got and make sure it lasts.

Step 2: So how'd ya do? **Write a short reflection in your course journal.**

If the questionnaire indicated that your belief in your medicine is high, reflect on how that plays into your adherence.

If it's low, explore more fully what some of your concerns are. Are they rooted in big pharma in general? Is it the specific medication? Is it your doctor, whom you suspect is pill-happy?

Tip 1: Don't fret if you scored low on the questionnaire. Low belief in medication is very common. We'll address ways to deal with it in future sessions.

Tip 2: If this session suggests to you that you are unconvinced about your treatment plan, schedule an appointment with your doctor to discuss it and perhaps think of alternatives.

Tip 3: Gain more clarity of what you do and do not believe in by checking out our Cultivating Authenticity course.

I'm glad that you've decided to join us for the Adhering to Your Medication course. Each session of our course consists of a warm-up talk, followed by a hands-on component where you'll learn a new skill or idea and have a chance to start putting it into action.

We're going to start the course by taking a fundamental look at what psychologists call our core beliefs.

In the talk we're about to watch, Dr. Lauren Hazzouri explains how core beliefs guide our behaviors. You'll be surprised at the impact you can have on your life by simply slowing down and identifying your beliefs. As you watch, think about how your core beliefs impact how adherent you tend to be with your medications.

(Plus: Check out our Defining Your Identity course 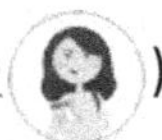)

We think you'll find that the more you put into the course, the more you'll get out of it. So take full advantage of all our features and find your place in a community of people facing similar challenges.

Enjoy!

Watch 'Core Beliefs' presented by Dr. Lauren Hazzouri on YouTube.

Does belief have anything to do with medication adherence?

Life isn't a J.M. Barrie novel. Clapping and believing in my meds won't make them work any better. Will it?

For:

1. There is no relationship between adherence and belief in my meds. I simply forget. End of story.
2. I believe that some medicine works some of the time, but what can I do that it actually doesn't work on me? It's not a question of belief; it's fact.
3. Things still come up all the time, even for people who believe in their meds 100 percent. Belief doesn't provide a buffer for life's daily distractions!

Add your own argument:

4. ____

Against:

1. Actually, according to research, there *is* a psychological factor to adherence that has to do with belief. The more belief you have in the necessity and safety of medication plan, the better chances you have of actually following through.
2. In terms of your general belief in phenomena as a person, you're probably right. You can be a very skeptical type who is super adherent. We're talking about a specific type of belief – confidence in your *ability* to follow the medical rules.
3. The more confident you are in your ability to adhere, the greater your chances of adherence!

Add your own argument:

4. ____

Medication beliefs strongly affect individuals' management of chronic diseases, expert says

Nearly half of patients taking medications for chronic conditions do not strictly follow their prescribed medication regimens. Failure to use medications as directed increases patients' risk for side effects, hospitalizations, reduced quality of life and shortened lifespans. Now, a University of Missouri gerontological nursing expert says patients' poor adherence to prescribed medication regimens is connected to their beliefs about the necessity of prescriptions and concerns about long-term effects and dependency.

MU Assistant Professor Todd Ruppar found that patients' beliefs about the causes of high blood pressure and the effectiveness of treatment alternatives significantly affected their likelihood of faithfully following prescribed medication regimens. In his pilot study, Ruppar focused on older patients' adherence to medication treatments that control high blood pressure, a condition that affects nearly 70 million adults in the U.S. and can lead to heart disease and stroke.

"Often, patients with chronic diseases are prescribed medications but they already have underlying beliefs about the causes of high blood pressure and how it can be treated, which leads them to underuse their medications," Ruppar said. "For example, some individuals might be able to reduce their blood pressure by walking or cutting down on salt consumption; however, most people need medication to reduce their risk of adverse health outcomes."

Rather than relying on education approaches, Ruppar says practitioners should aim to amend patients' behaviors using tactics such as electronic pill bottle caps that alert patients to take medications at specific times or more frequent monitoring of their blood pressure levels so they associate medication adherence with health benefits and non-adherence with negative side effects.

"Patients benefit from objective feedback to see what led them to miss doses, such as varying sleep patterns or weekend schedules. Then, they can change their routines to make taking doses as habitual as brushing their teeth," Ruppar said. "Self-management is important because encounters with health care providers are fairly short, so as patients, we tend to have better outcomes if we work with our providers to manage our chronic conditions."

The study, "Medication Beliefs and Antihypertensive Adherence Among Older Adults: A Pilot Study," was published in Geriatric Nursing. Ruppar is an assistant professor and the John A. Hartford Foundation and Atlantic Philanthropies Claire M. Fagin Fellow in the MU Sinclair School of Nursing. Ruppar's coauthors include Fabienne Dobbels, an assistant professor at the University of Leuven in Belgium, and Sabina De Geest, a professor at the University of Leuven and the University of Basel in Switzerland.

From ScienceDaily

I don't believe in my meds and here's why

If you don't believe in your medication, there is really very little motivating you to put yourself out in order to take them consistently. Spend a few minutes thinking why you don't believe in your medication, and perhaps gain some insight as to why you should give it a chance.

Take some time brainstorming in your journal about your experience with your medication, and then share your story with the Buddy and Soul community! Direct message us YOUR story @Buddy_N_Soul on Instagram and be anonymously featured for a chance to **win a Buddy&Soul three month free membership**. You can also tag us on Instagram and Twitter @Buddy_N_Soul, using the **#BuddynSoulMedSupport**. By sharing with us on social media, not only can you help others with their personal journeys, you can read about those facing similar challenges.

The core belief that was harming my adherence

Whether a distrust of doctors, or the loss of a loved one from a similar condition, it can often be a core belief that keeps us from adhering to our medication. Have you recognized a core belief that was holding you back? Share with the community and maybe gain some insight regarding the belief, and help others who are facing similar challenges.

Direct message us YOUR story @Buddy_N_Soul on Instagram and be anonymously featured for a chance to **win a Buddy&Soul three month free membership**.

Did you know that, Dr. Colleen McHorney's 2009 study *The Adherence Estimator* rated **patient knowledge** (along with patient trust and medication-safety) as one of the big three determinants of how consistent you'll be about following your treatment plan?

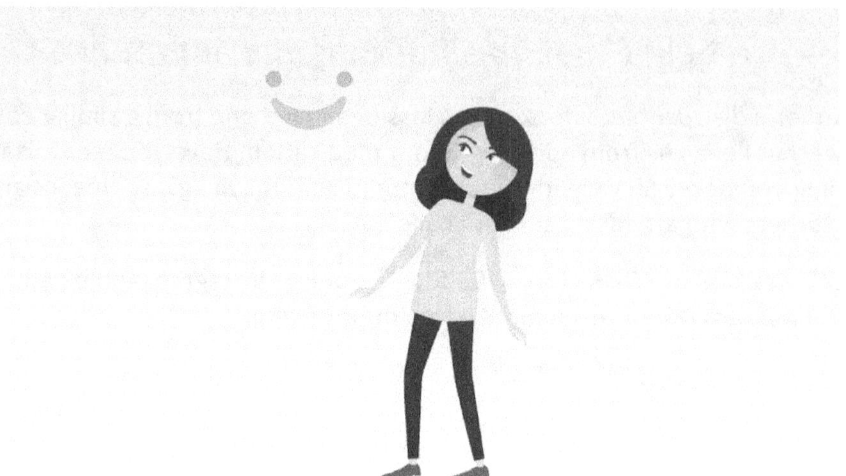

If you're already pretty informed about the medication you're on, that's great! If not, schedule some time for yourself to read up or speak with knowledgeable individuals to increase your expertise about your medication.

Your doctor is obviously a great source of information, and if you can learn from her, it's wonderful. But she does not have to be your only source of information. Reach out to those around you who can help you get the info you need.

Some questions to consider are:

- Why your doctor may have prescribed this particular medication
- What the alternatives are, and whether there is a significant cost and efficacy difference between them
- How it works on the technical-medical level
- How easy is it to take, and how often you have to take it
- Possible side effects
- How immediately you'll see results from your medication
- Anything else you might want to know

Some of these elements can be big deterrents to adherence.

Strengthen your ability to adhere by upping your knowledge-base. Because the more you know, the more power you will have in this journey, and the greater the chances you'll successfully adhere to your treatment.

Additionally, the more you know, the greater the possibility to be involved in choosing, alongside your doctor, your treatment course.

Academic research on shared decision-making has shown that when patients take an active role in choosing their treatment course, they are more likely to adhere to it. So go out and get knowledgeable!

EXERCISE

Step 1: Take this single-item survey:

How knowledgeable are you about your medication?

Step 2: **Identify what more you'd need to find out to bring your score closer to a 5.**

For example, consider why your doctor prescribed your particular medication, what the alternatives are, how it works medically, and so forth.

TIPS

Tip 1: Schedule some time into your calendar to research and fill in the information gaps. It doesn't have to be a huge block of time. Just get it done. Commit to it and follow through.

Tip 2: To make sure you understand the info you got, try to explain what you learned to a friend or family member. You can record the explanation.

Tip 3: Some companies, like Treato, gather patient feedback about medication. See what they have to say about yours.

Tip 4: Feel free to use your Buddy&Soul journal for reference as you maneuver your way through the course and through improving your medication adherence.

Tip 5: If anything surprising comes to your attention, make sure to bring it up with your doctor right away!

Hi, and welcome to the next session of our book. We're glad you've returned and we look forward to deepening our understanding of medication adherence. Let's get started!

There's a lot of discussion today about patient-centered medicine versus doctor-centered medicine. Is the expertise flowing from the healthcare system to the patient? Or from the patient to the health-care system? Roni Zeiger, M.D., left his position as the former Chief Health Strategist at Google, and founded with Gilles Frydman 'Smart Patients,' in order to amplify the knowledge created by networks of engaged patients.

In this talk, Zeiger will give several examples of how patients, who have become experts in the science of their disease, have banded together through thoughtful collaboration, and made huge advances in their disease. In his words, "we are a network of 'micro-experts,'" and we need to utilize the information that we have in order to better others and ourselves.

Watch 'Who is the Real Medical Expert' presented Roni Zeiger on YouTube.

9 Reasons knowledge is power when it comes to your meds

Research shows that the more you know about your meds, the more likely you are to take them properly. Here are some reasons why.

1. Flexibility. The more you know about your meds, the greater flexibility you will have with your adherence. Instead of throwing in the towel if you miss a dose, you'll know exactly what your next step should be. Rest assured you're not the first person to have missed a dose!
2. Motivation. It's easy to lose sight of the fact that your medication is helping you, especially if it offers no immediate gains. The less you view your medication as some mystical magic potion, the more motivated you'll be to adhere.
3. Resilience. If your treatment plan doesn't seem to be working, it's easy to blame the physician. Instead, get informed about the various alternative options. If you understand why this med was chosen, or better yet, if you were involved in the decision yourself, you're likely to be much more proactive about finding solutions and alternatives.

   (Plus: Check out our Manage Your Medical Condition and Emotionally Manage Your Illness courses)

4. Sense of control. When it comes to illness and medication, it's disheartening when you feel as though everything is being done to you, for you, and on your behalf. Becoming actively involved in the medical decision-making process empowers you by granting you a sense of control. And that begins with getting informed.
5. Knowing when to speak up. You are the number one sounding board for your physician. They might know the inner workings of the body better than you do, but only you know how your particular body is reacting to this particular medication option. A highly informed patient will know which symptoms and side effects require further attention and which they can just let slide.
6. Critical thinking. Being a good doctor requires skill and years of practice. Well, guess what... so does being a good patient! If you're informed about your medical condition and about your medications, you'll know if something doesn't quite sound right. You might ask further questions or pursue a second opinion. But without the proper knowledge base, you'll never have the confidence to think critically about the treatment you're receiving.

Add your own:

7. ____

8. ____

9. ____

Does knowledge increase adherence to meds?

Education is the usual go-to for changing behavior. And yet we still find no shortage of smokers, drunk drivers, or people engaging in unsafe sex who know full well what the ramifications of their choices may be. So, what's to say that if I knew more about my meds I would be any better at sticking to them? (Plus: **Check out our** Tackling Change course)

For:

1. Of course it does. The more I know, the more my knowledge influences my behavior.
2. I'm convinced that if someone would take the time to explain the medical basis that underlies my treatment, my adherence would be forever improved.
3. Humans can think things through. Our neocortex sets us apart from animals. Let's use it!

Add your own argument:

4. ____

Against:

1. Knowledge is important, yes. But at the end of the day, I prefer to go with my gut instinct.
2. I know I should take my meds properly, and I don't. More knowledge would simply lead to more contradictory behavior. I'm not proud of it, but c'est la vie.
3. What about all the emotional richness we all possess? I, for one, am more motivated by the emotional ramifications of being unwell than by facts and figures. There is more to sticking to my plan than knowledge.

Add your own argument:

4. ____

How learning about my treatment helped me improve my adherence

Share with the community how knowledge and education helped you overcome your difficulties with medication adherence. Inspire others to go the extra mile and learn more about their treatment as well.

Take some time brainstorming in your journal about your experience with your medication, and then share your story with the Buddy and Soul community! Tag us on Instagram and Twitter @Buddy_N_Soul, using the **#BuddynSoulMedSupport**. You can also direct message us YOUR story @Buddy_N_Soul on Instagram and be anonymously featured for a chance to **win a Buddy&Soul three month free membership**. By sharing with us on social media, not only can you help others with their personal journeys, you can read about those facing similar challenges.

How I got inspired to become an expert on my illness

Even if you trust your doctors implicitly, there is immense value in becoming an educated expert on your own medical needs and medications. Share with the community how Zeiger inspired you to become a micro-expert, and how it affected your adherence to your medication.

Direct message us YOUR story @Buddy_N_Soul on Instagram and be anonymously featured for a chance to **win a Buddy&Soul three month free membership**. By sharing with us on social media, not only can you help others with their personal journeys, you can read about those facing similar challenges.

Strategy 3: Finding the missing factor

Why on earth would someone not be 1000% adherent to their medication? Well, if you've been on medication for a while, you know the answer is 'it's complicated.' You and only you have a chance of figuring out why this happens to you. And we will help you figure out why.

When a doctor prescribes a medication or treatment plan she usually focuses on the drug's medical benefits. This is obviously the primary concern, since you're not going to take medication that doesn't offer you a medical benefit. And yet, **doctors sometimes ignore other seemingly insignificant aspects that are actually quite critical when it comes to adherence to medication.**

A study from the Tuck School of Business at Dartmouth College demonstrated how the following factors (or lack thereof) contributed to adherence:

- How immediately you can see the results of your meds (take my meds ⬜ don't have pain).
- How easy the medication is to take.
- How much you have to pay out-of-pocket.
- The existence and intensity of side effects – both in terms of their frequency and severity.

Does any of the above sound familiar to you?

Other factors might be:

- To what extent you feel informed and involved in the decision-making process.
- Cultural factors, like stigma associated with your illness.
- How well the medication works with your lifestyle.

Do one or more of these factors influence how you adhere to your medication? If so, you are not alone. The Exercise component that follows will address the above factors and others that may be hindering your adherence to your medication.

Step 1: What gets in the way of optimal adherence to your treatment?
Note your answers in your journal.

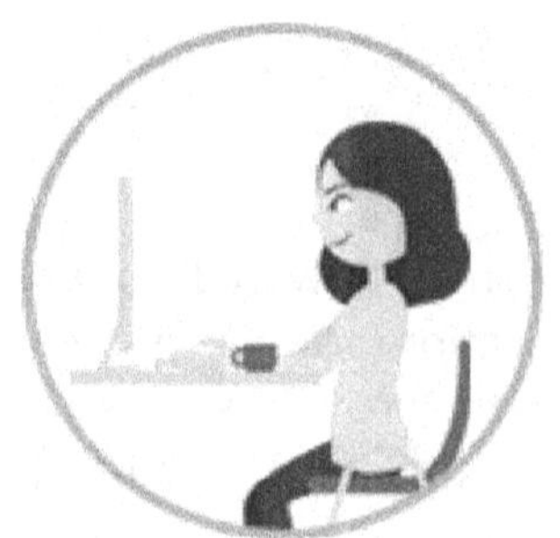

1. I don't think my meds work.
2. The medication is hard to take.
3. My meds are costly.
4. Taking my meds interferes with my lifestyle.
5. The medication takes too long to kick in initially.
6. The side effects bother me.
7. I don't feel a part of my treatment plan, so why bother?
8. The stigma involved with being labeled "a patient".
9. Anger! I don't want to be ill.

Step 2: Write a letter to someone you love convincing them to adhere to their meds despite the challenge involved.

Consider the answers you rated the highest. Now imagine your child, partner, or very close friend confiding in you that they weren't adhering to their meds for those very reasons. What would you tell them that would validate their struggle and help guide them in the right direction?

TIPS

Tip 1: Keep the factors that most bother you in mind as you progress through the sessions of the course, and learn how to deal with them effectively.

Tip 2: Are you looking for a way to change how you think and feel about your meds? Be sure to check out our Everyday Reframing course. 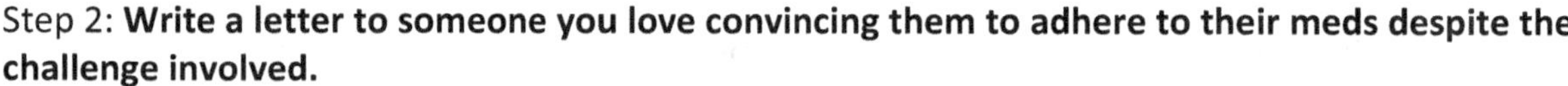

Today's session is going to have you questioning what hold you back from optimal adherence. Or in other words, why do so many of us find it so challenging to take our meds?

In the warm-up talk we're about to watch, psychologist Barry Schwartz talks about the paradox of choice. And how, sadly, the more choices we have, the more unhappy we become.
As you're watching think about how your own adherence would look if you knew there was just one option available to you.

Watch 'The Paradox of Choice' presented by Barry Schwartz on YouTube.

Is there always a deeper reason people struggle with adherence?

Sure, you can always dig deep and find legitimate excuses for why people struggle with adherence. But when it comes down to the honest truth, most people aren't adhering to their meds simply because they don't want to. No need to look any further than that!

For:

1. I'd like to believe the simple equation of I want = I do, I don't want = I don't do. The thing is that life is just not that simple.
2. When you're an adult, sometimes you have to do things that are hard, annoying, unpleasant... It's a red flag if an adult can't pull it together.
3. There is no one who wants to sabotage their own health. There must be something deeper going on.

Add your own argument:

4. ____

Against:

1. Sometimes people – even responsible, capable adults – just can't be bothered to take their meds. The end.
2. For some people, poor compliance comes down to simple things like pill size, the inconvenience of refilling prescriptions, and simple forgetfulness.
3. Sure there are those who struggle with adherence on a deeper, more fundamental level, but who says they are the rule and not the exception?

Add your own argument:

4. ____

3 Adherence hacks for adventurous types

Medication adherence is challenging for *everyone*. No matter how much you thrive on consistency and routines, somehow it's different with your meds. And for those of us who like to be spontaneous and fly by the seat of our pants? Well, adherence just requires that much more effort. Here are a few adherence challenges – and possible solutions – for patients with more adventurous natures.

(Plus: Check out our Defining Your Identity and Cultivating Authenticity courses 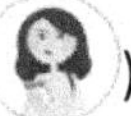)

1. The challenge: Routines. You *hate* them. Doing the same thing every day makes you feel like you're in jail.

A solution: Create variety where you can. If it's a daily med, at least try varying where you are when you take it, or how you do it (while singing your favorite song from *The Sound of Music*, for instance).

2. The challenge: Organization is not your strong suit. You have missed appointments and forgotten to pick up your meds on time simply because you had no calendar or reminder system set up.

A solution: Download a reminder app or buy a mini pen-and-paper planner and put it in your bag today. Before you leave any appointment, book your next one and pledge not to leave that office without marking it down. Same idea for picking up your meds from the pharmacy.

3. The challenge: Since boredom is the enemy of adventurous types, you like to fill your time and keep yourself on the go. This sometimes leads to missed medication dosages. Oops.

A solution: Plan for spontaneity (seriously). There's no need to sit at home all day, waiting for your medication alarm to sound. By all means, keep up your busy life! Just make sure you have a plan B in case you don't get home on time for your meds.

Can you think of a challenge that you may face and plan a possible solution? Write it in your journal.

The missing factor that hindered my medication adherence

Taking your meds on time seems like an easy and obvious thing to do — until you're the one required to do it. Adherence is a problem for a great many people, but it's a different thing holding each person back from perfect adherence. So what was your missing factor? What was the broken link that was stopping you from taking your meds like you knew you should?

Direct message us YOUR story @Buddy_N_Soul on Instagram and be anonymously featured for a chance to **win a Buddy&Soul three month free membership**.

10 Surprising ideas about choice

In his TED Talk *The Paradox of Choice,* Barry Schwartz introduces concepts that throw popular notions like the empowering nature of choice and decision-making out the window. Considering all the medication options out there, it's worth considering what all this means for our health.

1. More choice does not equal more freedom. In fact, it equals paralysis.
2. Patient autonomy can be negative when you shift responsibility from the doctor who is informed and knowledgeable to the patient who is sick and not necessarily in the best shape to make decisions.
3. People can accomplish less in their lives than in the past because they are preoccupied with making important choices.
4. Almost everything in life is a choice nowadays. That's a whole lot of choice!
5. Too much choice almost inevitably ends in being unhappy with the choice that was made. Think about it, there's always another option, or another option, or another option to have doubts about.
6. Too much choice means constantly living with a fear of missing out.
7. With every choice our expectations get higher and higher.

Add your own:

8. ____

9. ____

10. ____

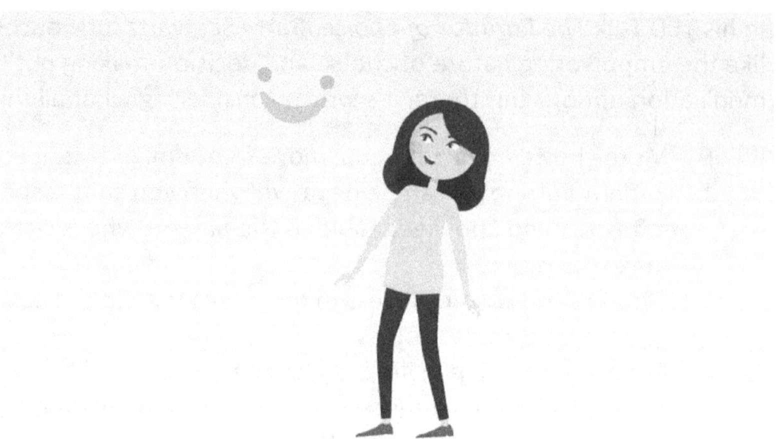

Sometimes what stops us from being adherent to our medication is deeper than just forgetfulness, disliking our doctor, or the bitter taste of the pill.

For example, would you believe that according to a study, nearly a quarter of those who have undergone kidney transplants do not adhere to their medication simply because they are tired of being told what to do?

Emotional probing can easily reveal a plethora of associations, past challenges, traumas, or other issues that might impact how consistently you will follow your medical regimen. In the previous session we addressed what might be holding you back, and knowing is half the battle. The other half is checking that baggage at the door.

Have you ever considered what stigmas you may be fighting by not wanting to be 'sick?' The fear you may be facing by admitting you are no longer young, healthy, perfect, or invincible? The desperate need to be in control of something you can no longer control?

These are just some of the many emotional rollercoasters you may be experiencing when you think about your medication. Or maybe you're really just forgetful—but it's worth taking the time to figure out which option is true to your reality.

If you suspect that any of the above may factor into your adherence, worry not; you can start dealing with this baggage in the comfort of your own space, right now, by turning an honest eye (and ear) inwards.

For every negative factor, belief, or influence holding you back from adherence to your meds exists a positive spin—what is called a "reframe" in professional psychological language. You have the power to take a negative emotion or fear and reframe it as something better.

For example, maybe you don't adhere because someone you were close to had a similar condition and the meds didn't help them. You're angry at that and don't fully trust your treatment.

But instead of saying *"I don't trust my medication,"* you can say, "M*edicine is changing every day, and each person is different. My loved one would want me to do everything in my power to keep myself well, even if it didn't work for them."*

The facts are the same, but the emotion of distrust isn't dismissed. It's just viewed through a different prism.

(Plus: Check out our Everyday Reframing course 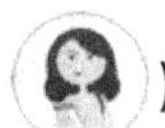)

EXERCISE

Step 1: Use your journal to **list some thoughts that have a negative impact on your adherence.**

These might be things that are holding you back or ideas that are stalling or weakening your resolve.

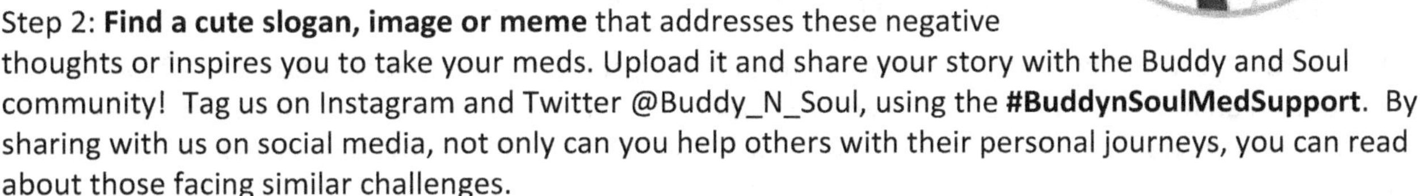

Step 2: **Find a cute slogan, image or meme** that addresses these negative thoughts or inspires you to take your meds. Upload it and share your story with the Buddy and Soul community! Tag us on Instagram and Twitter @Buddy_N_Soul, using the **#BuddynSoulMedSupport**. By sharing with us on social media, not only can you help others with their personal journeys, you can read about those facing similar challenges.

TIPS

Tip 1: Sometimes airing your negative emotions is enough. However, if you need more help to deal with what comes out in your quiet meditation or brainstorming, it might be time to take action and reach out for help.

Tip 2: Reluctant to share your feelings with anyone? Try just spelling out your medication-related emotional baggage to yourself. It's is already a big step toward dealing with it.

Tip 3: Some might find it easier to meditate shortly (on their medical condition, their medicine and their adherence) before beginning or in order to spark future reflection.

Tip 4: Use this as your jumping board to encourage further inner-dialogue and deeper internal digging. For more tools on how to identify and explore your feelings check out our Emotionally Manage Your Illness course.

DRIVING THE MESSAGE HOME

Hi, and thank you for joining us for the next session, and for having what it takes to really tackle medication adherence.

So… what do you call a veterinarian who can only take care of one species? A physician!

In a fascinating talk, Barbara Natterson-Horowitz shares how a species-spanning approach to health can improve medical care — particularly when it comes to mental health.

In her words, "veterinarians had been diagnosing, treating and even preventing emotionally induced symptoms in animals ranging from monkeys to flamingos, from to deer to rabbits, since the 1970s." And yet, doctors have not made the cross-over between what we can learn from animals and deduce to humans.

When it comes to knowing yourself and how you adhere to your medication, your emotional baggage may be playing a central part. It's important to identify your feelings, and how they may be influencing your adherence.

We hope you enjoy this thought-provoking talk!

Watch 'What Veterinarians Know That Doctors Don't' presented by Barbara Natterson-Horowitz on YouTube.

9 Emotions that stop you from adhering to your medication

If you felt totally fine with taking your meds, you'd probably be taking them, no problem. And if you felt totally fine not taking your meds, you wouldn't be taking them at all, and would have no problem telling your doctor that you're not.

If you find yourself not taking your meds and not talking to your doctor about it, there could be something else going on.

(Plus: Check out our Emotionally Manage Your Illness course 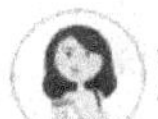)

1. Shame. There must be something wrong with me that I need to take medication.
2. Embarrassment. Not to be mistaken for shame, embarrassment is that experience you get when someone else catches you doing something wrong. It's embarrassing to think that you are sick and need meds.
3. Anger. I'm mad at my doctor. I'm mad at myself. I'm mad at the world. And definitely too mad to take my meds.
4. Guilt. I know I should be taking my meds and I'm not. If something happens to me, it'll be my fault.
5. Sadness. I can't get past this internal voice reminding me I'm no longer invincible. I mourn the good old days, when I was healthy.
6. Denial. It's okay if I skip a dose every now and again…isn't it?

Add your own:

7. ____

8. ____

9. ____

Depression associated with poor medication adherence in patients with chronic illnesses

People who are depressed are less likely to adhere to medications for their chronic health problems than patients who are not depressed, putting them at increased risk of poor health, according to a new RAND Corporation study.

Researchers found that depressed patients across a wide array of chronic illnesses such as diabetes and heart disease had 76 percent greater odds of being non-adherent with their medications compared to patients who were not depressed. The findings were published online by the Journal of General Internal Medicine.

The study is the largest systematic review to date to look at the role that depression plays in medication adherence among patients in the United States.

"These findings provide the best evidence to date that depression is an important risk factor that may influence whether patients adhere to their medications," said Dr. Walid F. Gellad, the study's senior author and a natural scientist at RAND, a nonprofit research organization. "There are important implications for both patient health and for health care costs.

"Doctors and other providers should periodically ask patients with depression about medication adherence. Also, when treating a patient who is not taking their medication correctly, they should consider the possibility that depression is contributing to the problem."

Poor adherence to prescribed medication is a well-known problem that is associated with higher death rates among people with chronic illnesses. It is also blamed for increasing U.S. health care costs.

Researchers from RAND and the Claremont Graduate School conducted the study by examining past studies that have measured medication adherence. They combined information from 31 studies involving more than 18,000 people -- significantly more than past reviews -to examine the link between medication adherence and depression.

The study is the first to review the association between depression and medication adherence for patients with high blood pressure and high cholesterol. Other conditions examined in the study include coronary heart disease, diabetes and asthma. The link between depression and medication adherence did not vary significantly between the different chronic illnesses, said Gellad, who is also a physician with the VA Pittsburgh Healthcare System.

"The consistent link between depression and nonadherence across all these illnesses underscores the seriousness of the role that depression plays in keeping people from properly managing chronic conditions," said Jerry L. Grenard, the study's lead author and an assistant professor at the Claremont Graduate School. "That consistency also suggests that lessons learned about how to improve medication adherence among depressed patients with one disease may be applied to other chronic conditions."

Researchers say that depression is just one barrier to getting patients to follow medication recommendations. Additional well-documented barriers to medication adherence are dose complexity and patient cost-sharing. Other barriers that may play a role include beliefs about medications, social support, side effects and provider factors.

The study was supported by the Agency for Healthcare Research and Quality and by Mehlman Vogel Castagnetti.

Other authors of the study are Brett A. Munjas, John L. Adams, Marika Suttorp and Margaret Maglione of RAND, and Elizabeth A. McGlynn of Kaiser Permanente.

From ScienceDaily

My biggest obstacle when adhering to my medication

While there are a lot of reasons out there to be less-than-perfectly-adherent to your medication, most of us have one big obstacle that holds us back. What is your biggest setback when it comes to your meds? Share with the community, and maybe learn a new trick or two for overcoming your own challenge while you're at it.

Take some time brainstorming in your journal about your experience with your medication, and then share your story with the Buddy and Soul community! Tag us on Instagram and Twitter @Buddy_N_Soul, using the **#BuddynSoulMedSupport**. You can also direct message us YOUR story @Buddy_N_Soul on Instagram and be anonymously featured for a chance to **win a Buddy&Soul three month free membership**. By sharing with us on social media, not only can you help others with their personal journeys, you can read about those facing similar challenges.

Should physicians take their cues from veterinarians?

In a fascinating TED Talk, Barbara Natterson-Horowitz suggests that the medical community adopt a species-spanning approach, particularly in the field of mental health. While it's a nice idea, surely humans are fundamentally different from animals. Would insights about animal care really improve human medical care?

For:

1. By and large, animals and humans suffer from the same illnesses and respond to the same treatments. It makes sense to cross-compare.
2. Most drugs are tested on animals before they reach your pharmacy. If we're similar enough to share drugs, we're similar enough to learn from one another's care.

Add your own argument:

3. ____

Against:

1. Humans and animals are absolutely distinct. It's offensive to suggest otherwise.
2. There is far greater expertise in human medicine than in veterinary medicine. Go where the research is stronger...and better funded.

Add your own argument:

3. ____

Strategy 5: What's your conscientiousness level?

Adherence to medication (or, to be honest, non-adherence) is a huge topic, and a frustrating one too, because it's so complicated. Finding one variable that would predict non-adherence would be a game-changer; psychologists Brent Roberts of the University of Illinois and Patrick Hill of Washington University have done just that.

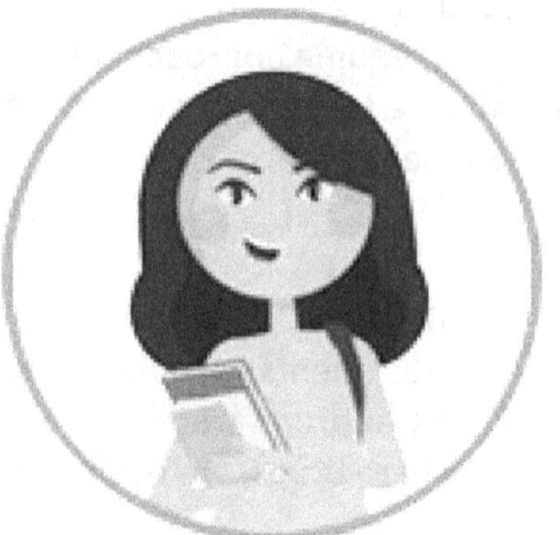

They defined 'conscientiousness' as the tendency to stick with rules and regimens. According to their findings, "conscientious individuals report higher levels of both doctor and medication adherence."

Some folks are super conscientious. My mom is one of them. Following a hip joint surgery, she had to do physical therapy exercises at home. When I visited, I would see her do ten of each. At the seventh it was evident she was in great pain. By the ninth she was crying. But none of it stopped her from completing all ten, as prescribed.

Are you like that? If so, then you are highly conscientious and probably only need to be working through this course to learn a few new tricks.

But not everyone is like my mom. Some of us are more prone to breaking rules, or shelving them – for an evening, a day, or as long as you feel like it.

I can guess what you're going to ask now. Since not everyone can be super-conscientious, why bother? Well, for starters, remember that it's not an all-or-nothing scenario. Conscientiousness is a scale, and even if you aren't at the high extreme, you likely still have what to work with. And if there's a medication you need to stick to, conscientiousness is important. So, figure out your conscientiousness level and take it from there.

Once you know how conscientious you are, you can start working with your natural tendencies to enhance your adherence levels.

If you're naturally highly conscientious, you're probably pretty adherent. You'll just need to watch out for the odd days here and there when you might get busy and forget. If you're naturally less conscientious, on the other hand, research show that good adherence will pose more of a challenge so you'll need to work a little harder.

Your level of conscientiousness is a lever, not an excuse. Use it to choose the tips and tricks (from the course here or from anywhere else) that will help you push your adherence higher. The end goal is that you feel better.

And without further ado, let's get right to it.

EXERCISE

Respond to the questionnaire below to figure out your level of consientiousness. Read each of the following statements and rate the level at which you agree on a scale of 1 to 4, with 1 being strongly disagree and 4 being strongly agree.

(Source: Based on Roberts, B. W., Walton, K. E., & Bogg, T. (2005). Conscientiousness and health across the life course. *Review of General Psychology, 9(2), 156.*)

A. I am easily talked into doing silly things.

B. I support long-established rules and traditions.

C. I rarely jump into something without first thinking about it.

D. I do not intend to follow every little rule that others make up.

E. I often rush into action without thinking about potential consequences.

F. Even if I knew how to get around the rules without breaking them, I would not do it.

G. I am careful what I say to others.

H. When I was in school, I used to break rules quite regularly.

Scorecard:

	What you ranked yourself:			
	1	2	3	4
Question #:	What it's worth:			
A.	4	3	2	1
B.	1	2	3	4
C.	1	2	3	4
D.	4	3	2	1
E.	4	3	2	1
F.	1	2	3	4
G.	1	2	3	4
H.	4	3	2	1
TOTAL:				

High 24-32 message: You scored high. This course is also perfect for you! Learn to understand your inner workings and what helps keep your adherence levels so high.

Medium 16-23 message: You got a medium score; you have work to do but you also have some natural strengths to work with.

Low 8-15 message: Your conscientiousness level is low. But don't be discouraged by a low score. This course is here to help you address the problem areas and maximize your adherence.

TIPS

Tip 1: If you're low on conscientiousness, you might want to also practice Buddy&Soul's Willpower 101 course to help you stick to your medication regimen. 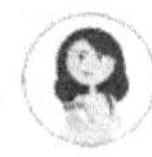

Tip 2: If you're high on conscientiousness check out our Habit Workshop course 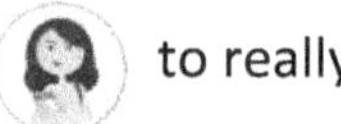 to really maximize your medication regimen.

Tip 3: Your conscientiousness level should help guide your adherence efforts. The lower you are, the more help you'll need, and the more committed you'll have to decide to be. But – it's worth it!

Hey, we're happy to welcome you back to the next session of our course! We hope you like the clip we've selected for today's session.

Conscientiousness is considered one of the 'Big Five' personality traits according to personality psychology. By looking at a person's level of conscientiousness, along with openness, agreeableness, extraversion and emotional range, you can gain a very detailed understanding of a person.

When it comes to adherence to medication, these traits become a crucial part of understanding how well you naturally stick to medication, and how you can best go about improving your adherence.

Brian Little is a personality psychologist. In this talk you will hear him talk about the 'Big Five,' or the OCEAN (Open to experience, Conscientiousness, Extroversion, Agreeable individuals, Neurotic individuals). This will help you gain a better understanding of your personality and conscientiousness level.

If conscientiousness comes naturally for you, then adherence will be easier. However, if conscientiousness is less natural, you'll have to work a little bit harder to keep up that treatment plan.

Enjoy!

Watch 'Who Are You, Really? The Puzzle of Personality' presented by Brian Little on YouTube.

Should I bother working on adherence if I know I'm never gonna change?

There are those who say adherence is a skill you're born, and there are those who say it can be learned. Either way, is there really any point in working on something if it feels foreign and out of your comfort zone?

For:

1. Adherence is a skill. When I was born, I didn't know how to read or tie my shoes. And look at me now!
2. It's all about willpower and the mind. If I believe I can be perfectly compliant, I can be.
3. If my doctor prescribed a daily scoop of ice cream at 8 pm every night, I bet my "old dog" would learn that "new trick" in record time! I'll just make believe I enjoy taking my medications as much I love eating ice cream.

4. There's a sense of accomplishment in knowing I made a change. I'll use that for self-leverage.

Add your own argument:

5. ____

Against:

1. I wasn't born with an adherent nature. Why invest effort and energy into something that's a lost cause?
2. I think learning to accept myself as I am is more important for my health in the long run.
3. Just *thinking* of change gives me the jitters.

Add your own argument:

4. ____

6 Adherence struggles for not-so-conscientious types

When it comes to adherence to medication, we'd all love to be a Rabbit: super-conscientious, meticulous, and consistent to the point of slight absurdity. If it means we're taking our meds seriously, it might be worth it.

But we're not all wired that way (and thankfully so!). Lots of us are distractible Pooh-Bears, or excitable Tiggers, or slightly scatter-minded Piglets. Here are some common struggles that the non-conscientious are faced with when it comes to taking their meds.
(Plus: Check out our Defining Your Identity and Cultivating Authenticity courses 😊)

1. I'm happy with my not-so-perfect adherence! It's hard to push myself for more.
2. I like to operate quickly and efficiently. This can mean making decisions without my adherence in mind.
3. I am not a rule person, and I never will be. Tell me I got to take my meds and I'll show you!

Add your own:

4. ____

5. ____

6. ____

3 Reasons adherence is tough, even for conscientious folks

If you're a highly conscientious type, chances are you're pretty good about taking your meds properly. But that doesn't mean it comes easily! Here are a few reasons adherence would be tough even for the conscientiousness poster child.

1. Conscientiousness is a personality trait, nothing more. It doesn't drive to the drug store to pick up my meds for me. I still have to do all the leg work that any non-conscientious person would have to do.
2. My conscientiousness doesn't shield me from being human. No matter how much I believe in taking my meds properly, I still have days when I'm up against feeling exhausted, overwhelmed, depressed, and in despair.
3. Being highly conscientious means that if I do, heaven forbid, miss a pill one day, I berate myself for weeks – a challenge in and of itself!

Add your own:

4. ____

5. ____

6. ____

Why knowing about conscientiousness saved my adherence

Perhaps for the first time, I realized there wasn't something wrong with me, I was literally just wired for non-adherence. Surprisingly, that helped me adhere. Here's why.

Take some time brainstorming in your journal about your experience with your medication, and then share your story with the Buddy and Soul community! Tag us on Instagram and Twitter @Buddy_N_Soul, using the **#BuddynSoulMedSupport**. You can also direct message us YOUR story @Buddy_N_Soul on Instagram and be anonymously featured for a chance to **win a Buddy&Soul three month free membership**. By sharing with us on social media, not only can you help others with their personal journeys, you can read about those facing similar challenges.

My 'aha' about how my personality affects my adherence

We can tell you lots about personality and adherence, but only you can know how your personality affects your particular adherence patterns. Share with the community and help others who might be facing similar challenges and are looking for inspiration.

Direct message us YOUR story @Buddy_N_Soul on Instagram and be anonymously featured for a chance to **win a Buddy&Soul three month free membership**.

Your medical team, although well-trained in medicine, is not psychic.

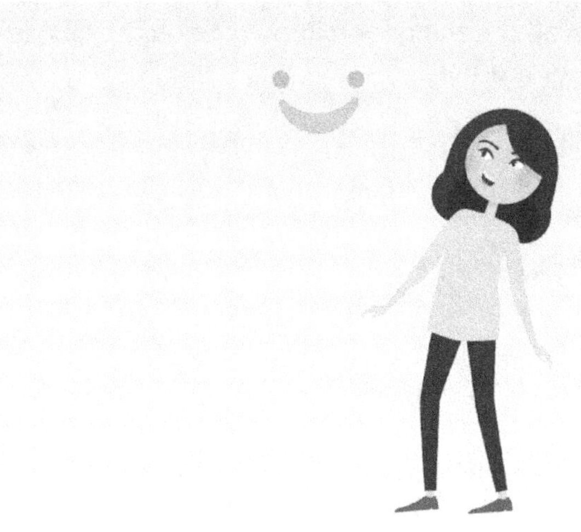

They have no idea what it's like to live in your body and feel your pain, discomfort, or improvement. This means that in order to build the greatest and most helpful relationship between you and your medical team, you need to include them in what's going on. Fill them in on your doubts about your medication and fess up to what you do and don't do when you're not in the doctor's office, even if it's embarrassing.

Most patients do not adhere to their medication 100% of the time, and yet, most patients do not report this to their medical team. By withholding valuable information from those who want and are most able to help, you are preventing yourself from getting the treatment you deserve.

Have you ever discussed non-adherence with your physician? Have you ever mentioned that you sometimes forget, get mixed up, or decide to skip? Does your doctor know that you're really taking your meds just 75% of the time? You might be afraid he or she will be angry or even disappointed with you, but the main goal is to have an honest discussion that will promote your health.

So – fess up! And while you're at it, let your doctor know when a big change has occurred either in your condition or in your therapy.

The responsibility falls on you to initiate the conversation with your doctors about changes in your health, fears or concerns about your therapy, and, of course, your adherence.

Admitting your fears and your faults takes guts, but it's important for two reasons:

1. Deep down, you know that taking responsibility for your actions is an integral part of being an adult.
2. Your health is at stake. If you're having a problem with following your treatment plan, your physician needs to know. You don't want them to have a false picture of what's going on and treat you accordingly. You and your physician might also discuss the option of switching medications, depending on your personal circumstances.

If you're wondering why this never came up at your appointments, research has found that many patients fail to report their poor adherence simply because they are not asked.

And you know what? When you face your doctor and fess up, you may find that the backlash you were expecting isn't quite as bad as you feared. Doctors often have suggestions of how to help, having helped other non-adherent patients in the past (told you you're not the first!).

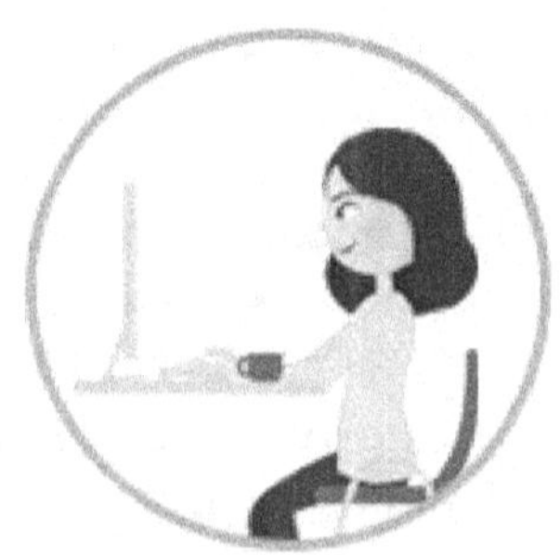

Step 1: **Write down all the things you know you ought to share with your medical team in your journal**.

Your updates, fears, concerns, struggles, new symptoms, and of course adherence to your medication. Keep it real!

Step 2: Ask yourself: what's the worst that can happen if you tell your doctor the things you just listed? Be specific: Will she smirk? And then what would happen? Will she make a nasty comment? And then what? Will she go on a shaming campaign on Facebook? Probably not. She'll likely just adjust your treatment and make a note in your file.

Keep going with the absolutely worst case-scenario, until you've reached a point where things can't possibly get worse. Are they as bad you feared?

TIPS

Tip 1: Admitting to vulnerability tends to be a relationship strengthener. So even though it might seem counterintuitive, being honest, even when you're horribly embarrassed, is more likely to boost your rapport than to damage it.

Tip 2: Don't be embarrassed about it. A lot of people aren't fully adherence to their meds. It's not what we're advocating, but that's life. So, be open and honest and help your physician help you figure it out.

Tip 3: When it comes time to ask your doctor, don't be shy! You can be sure they've been asked much weirder things in the course of their career.

Tip 4: Bring this list with you to your next appointment and share this important information with, and ask your questions of, your doctor. Ask about the ramifications of not taking your medication when you should and if there are alternatives that may fit your lifestyle better.

The healthcare industry in America is so focused on pathology, surgery, and pharmacology — on what doctors "do" to patients — that it often overlooks the values of the human beings it's supposed to care for.

Palliative care physician Timothy Ihrig explains the benefits of a different approach, one that fosters a patient's overall quality of life and navigates serious illness from diagnosis to death with dignity and compassion.

This is particularly relevant to our session which discusses the importance of being a team player with your doctors. However, in order to be a team with your doctors, your doctors have to be open to being team players as well. Doctors need to learn to engage the client where the client is at.

In Ihrig's words, "patient-centric care based on their values that helps this population live better and longer. It's a care model that tells the truth and engages one-on-one and meets people where they're at." So take some time to ensure that your medical team sees where you are at when it comes to your adherence. Together, you can make a treatment plan that is realistic and helpful for you.

Watch 'What We Can Do To Die Well' presented by Timothy Ihrig on YouTube.

Should I tell my doc I'm not adhering to my meds?

When it comes to taking my meds, I sometimes forget. Or don't want to. Or get busy. But is there really any point in sharing this with my doctor? I already know what I've got to do.

For:

1. My own integrity won't allow me to lie. I don't have to offer the info, but if doc asks, I will tell the truth.
2. Maybe there's something my physician can do to help me step up my game from now on. Maybe there's something she knows about that I don't.
3. My doctor treats me under the premise that I take my meds. If I don't take them and neglect to say this, my doctor may misinterpret my medical condition, prescribe more medication, or give a wrong diagnosis. Why would I hamper my medical treatment like this?

Add your own argument:

4. ____

Against:

1. There's no point. It's like if I tell my dentist I haven't flossed in the past 6 months – what's she gonna do about it now? If I lie, everyone's happy.
2. It's not what they mean when they ask. They just want to know that I'm basically doing fine with it, which I am. They aren't interested in all the nitty gritty details.
3. I don't want my physician to have an unfavorable impression of me. We have a really good rapport and I'd like to keep it that way.
4. Why waste the precious time? There are more important things I'd rather be discussing after waiting 8 months for this 15-minute appointment! Besides, I'm fairly certain I know what her thoughts will be on the matter.

Add your own argument:

5. ____

10 Reasons it's hard to be honest after not taking your meds

It's hard to share intimate information with people you don't feel so intimate with. And no matter how much you like or respect your physician, it's just not the same. So how can you bring yourself to share what you need to even without that sense of closeness?

(Plus: Check out our Cultivating Authenticity course 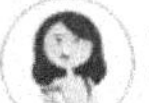)

1. Let's be honest, it's embarrassing. You know that you should know better. And needing to hear it from your doctor only makes it that much worse.
2. You don't want your doctor to be disappointed in you. You're supposed to be on the same team here. Still, if this is a real team, candor is key.
3. Hey, nobody's perfect, right? The doctor probably knows this and assumes you only take my meds part of the time. There's no need to tell her what she already knows! (Er, unless you want to get optimal treatment, that is.)
4. You don't want this knowledge to affect the quality of your future care. You might fear that if your doctor knew you weren't taking your meds properly then they may stop working as hard to help you.
5. You don't want to ruin the great relationship you've worked so hard to create. Then again, honesty is the bedrock of any relationship.
6. You feel bad and guilty that you haven't been doing your part, even when your physician has been doing his or hers. But don't forget — you're only human.
7. If your physician doesn't ask, it can't really be so important. On the other hand, appointments are so short...

Add your own:

8. ____

9. ____

10. ____

The moment I decided to stop faking my adherence

No one would ever know, not even your doctor. But you stopped faking adherence, anyway. So what was the moment you decided to stop faking, and owning up to your lack of adherence? What made you finally take responsibility for taking your meds?

Take some time brainstorming in your journal about your experience with your medication, and then share your story with the Buddy and Soul community! Direct message us YOUR story @Buddy_N_Soul on Instagram and be anonymously featured for a chance to **win a Buddy&Soul three month free membership**. You can also tag us on Instagram and Twitter @Buddy_N_Soul, using the **#BuddynSoulMedSupport**. By sharing with us on social media, not only can you help others with their personal journeys, you can read about those facing similar challenges.

5 Controversial insights about patient-centered care

Patient-centered care is a hot topic nowadays. Here are some provocative ideas inspired by Timothy Ihrig's TED Talk *What We Can Do to Die Well* that will get your mind thinking.

(Plus: Check out our Manage Your Medical Condition course 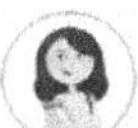)

1. Patient-centered care has been demonstrated to prolong patients' lives.
2. The focus is on truth, and not making the patient feel better.
3. The patients who have the most testing and treatments die earlier than those with fewer procedures.
4. Doctors deciding things can hinder the patient feeling as if they are living a life that they choose.
5. Patient-centered care is about living and not dying.

If you're like most people, you'll probably find that a tough time can be made easier by a little emotional support.

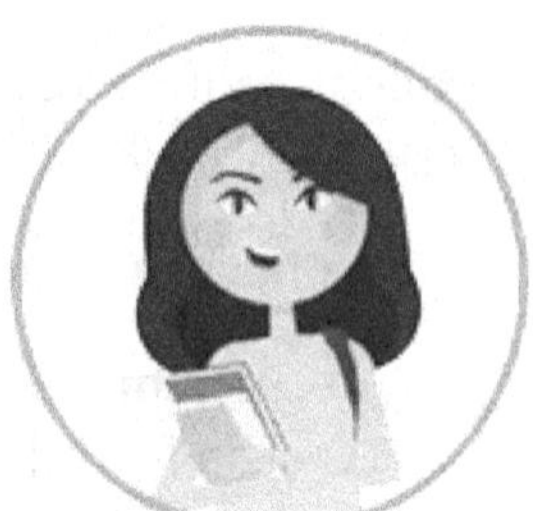

Support not only feels good, but actually has positive physiological effects, creating a healthier and stronger physical body.

Dr. David Spiegel, professor and associate chair of Psychiatry & Behavioral Sciences at Stanford University, discovered something ground-breaking in research from 1989 which is now a classic. Among women battling breast cancer, those who participated in support groups lived an average 18 months longer than those who did not.

When we share our struggles with others, especially others whom we feel really "get it," an amazing thing happens: we feel miraculously lighter, and in some amazing way, this affects our health.

Support comes in many forms. It can come, like in Spiegel's study, in the form of an official medical support group specific to your condition, which your physician might refer you to.

Nowadays, it might be a Facebook or Whatsapp group or some other social media community. Support can come in the form of regular conversations with a close friend, partner, family member, or someone else you know struggling with a long-term therapy.

Step 1: **Do a quick Google search for a support group**, either online or a local in-person option you might be willing to try.

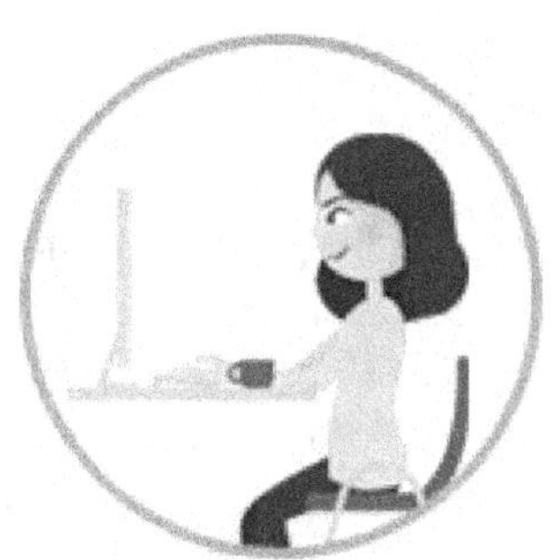

Save a screenshot of your search results so you'll have the information handy when you're ready to take the plunge.

Step 2: Make a time-based commitment to reach out to one of the support group options. It can be right now, later today, or later this week. Putting a time on it will help make it happen. Schedule it into your calendar now.

TIPS

Tip 1: Although a one-off ventilation session is great for blowing off some steam, the greatest benefits of a support system are experienced when you check in regularly.

Tip 2: Don't be shy. Call up a friend to schedule some mutually convenient face-to-face or phone time, speak to your physician's office about joining a patient support program, whatever best suit your lifestyle and preferences. Take it seriously. Make yourself a priority!

Tip 3: Being supported emotionally is important. Cognitive behavioral therapy also highlights the importance of practical steps to get you to perform the desired behavior.

Tip 4: Really not your thing? Maybe give it a try nonetheless, just once. You might find great value.

DRIVING THE MESSAGE HOME

Pamela Wible, M.D., is a family physician born into a family of physicians. Her parents warned her not to pursue medicine, but she followed her heart only to discover that to heal her patients she had to first heal her profession.

So she decided to lead a series of town hall meetings throughout Lane County, Oregon where she invited her community to design their own ideal clinic. Open since 2005, Dr. Wible's community clinic has sparked a movement in which citizens are designing ideal clinics nationwide.

Her model is taught in medical schools and featured in Harvard School of Public Health's Renegotiating Health Care, a text examining major trends in American healthcare.

Her work has helped remove unnecessary boundaries between patients and doctors and has created hundreds of 'ideal clinics' that patients themselves have designed. A safe place of wisdom, communication, relationships, and love. A place to be supported throughout your medical journey.

Do you know where the closest ideal clinic is for you?

Watch 'How to Get Naked with Your Doctor' presented by Dr. Pamela Wible at TEDxSalem on YouTube.

7 Tips for joining an online medical support group

Perhaps joining an online support group sounds like a fine plan, but with so many options out there, it can be hard to know where to begin! These tips should help you get a good start.

Start here! Check out Buddy&Soul's own Medical community for starters. This way you can get support and practice the courses together.

1. Get specific about your needs. Figuring out what kind of support would best suit you is step one. For example, do you want a forum where you can be anonymous, or post as yourself? Ask yourself some questions before you begin your search.
2. Court your suitors. Spend some time poking around the Internet before committing to any one support group or forum. Because any meaningful commitment is preceded by a period of courtship.
3. Introduce yourself. Regardless of what you've determined as your online identity, make sure to say a little about yourself and what you're looking for when you join. This is a great way to break the ice.
4. Be helpful where you can. When people recognize you (i.e. your avatar) as someone who supports others, they'll be more inclined to "be there" for you too.

Add your own:

5. ____

6. ____

7. ____

Which traits do you look for in your adherence support people?

There are so many well-intending people out there. Which character traits set apart those who can help us improve our medication compliance from those who can't?

1. **Altruism.** How much are they thinking about helping me vs. helping themselves?
2. **Caring.** How much do they care about me?
3. **Strong will.** How much do they challenge me to do better?
4. **Trust-worthiness.** Have they earned my trust over time?
5. **Emotional intelligence.** Do they make room for my emotions? Can they handle me?

What else do you look for?

6. ____

7. ____

8. ____

How support helped me improve my adherence

Whether you're a private type, or an invite-everyone-in type, support can be an invaluable tool when it comes to adherence. Share with the community how you got support, what type of support, and how it helped improve your adherence. Maybe you can even inspire someone who is on the fence about asking for or getting support.

Take some time brainstorming in your journal about your experience with your medication, and then share your story with the Buddy and Soul community! Tag us on Instagram and Twitter @Buddy_N_Soul, using the **#BuddynSoulMedSupport**. You can also direct message us YOUR story @Buddy_N_Soul on Instagram and be anonymously featured for a chance to **win a Buddy&Soul three month free membership**. By sharing with us on social media, not only can you help others with their personal journeys, you can read about those facing similar challenges.

How an 'ideal clinic' would help me see adherence differently

While you always knew you had to take your meds, there was something so routine about it that it became background noise. Share with the community how you were affected by Pamela Wilbe's talk, and how her concept of the 'ideal clinic' and changed your perception of adherence.

Direct message us YOUR story @Buddy_N_Soul on Instagram and be anonymously featured for a chance to **win a Buddy&Soul three month free membership**.

Now that you have taken a look at your core beliefs, thoughts, and feelings about your medication, it's time to work on your behavior.
Even the most gung-ho conscientious patients forget to take their meds every now and again. So how can you do better?
The first step to increasing your adherence to medication (especially if this is a long-term med) is to set up a no-fail reminder system that will help you when your memory fails.

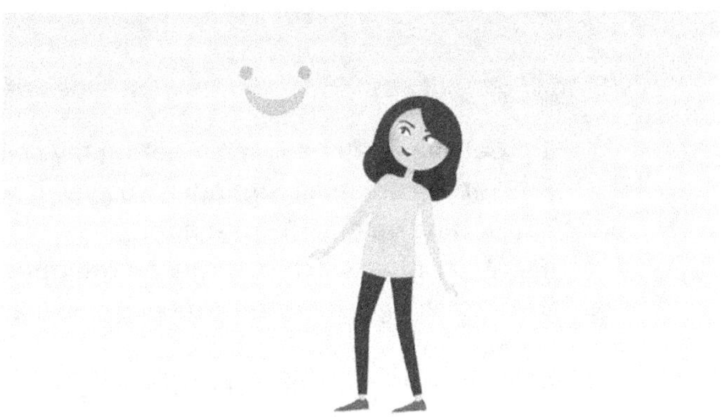

A reminder can be anything that works with your lifestyle – a phone alarm, a daily email alert, a pill alert app, a note in your day planner, a pre-arranged phone call from a friend, a discreet gesture from a partner, wearing your watch on your opposite wrist until you've taken your meds – the options are near-infinite!

Several studies, such as the one conducted by Kati Kannisto out of the University of Turko, have shown that a simple daily SMS reminder was enough to increase adherence when taking medications. This was true across a broad spectrum of sociodemographic backgrounds and various illness ranges. And even more successful than a 1-way text message reminder was a 2-way text message reminder, where the person responds back 'I did it'.

Reminders can be helpful not only for *taking* your meds, but also for *refilling your prescriptions on time.*

Warning: it's easier to botch this one than it seems.

Consider what happens if you're out of town or the pharmacy is closed by the time you swing by to collect your medication. Or how about if life gets busy and it simply slips your mind?

How are you going to plan ahead to make sure you always have your meds on hand when you need them?

Using reminders is definitely the easiest way to go, and can truly be a godsend.

Step 1: Would you find the following types of medication reminders helpful?

1. Setting a calendar reminder on my cell phone
2. Setting an email reminder, so I see it when I'm at my desk
3. Setting up an SMS reminder
4. Wearing a watch or a ring on the opposite hand every morning
5. Attaching it to an existing habit, like brushing my teeth or my afternoon coffee
6. Putting a physical note somewhere I'll see it—like on the medicine cabinet or inside my wallet
7. Downloading a medication reminder app

Step 2: Choose one of the options you chose as likely to be effective and commit to giving it a try ASAP. Write a pledge or commitment note here.

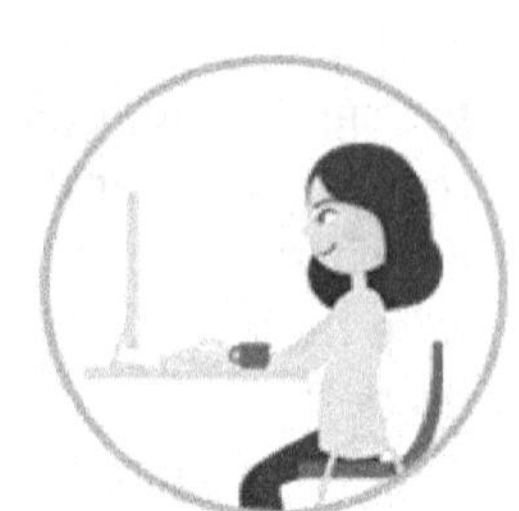

TIPS

Tip 1: If it's something you can do *right now*, do it! If you have to wait until you get home or are at the office, set a reminder to do it.

Tip 2: Remember—a reminder is just a tool; it can't replace your resolve or willpower to enhance your adherence to your medication! Be sure to check out our Willpower 101 course.

Tip 3: Be sure to give your reminder system a fair chance before you decide whether or not it's working well for you. You can always come back to your Buddy&Soul journal to jog your memory of some other medication reminder options.

Tip 4: For more on how to use reminders/triggers to your greatest benefit, check out our Habit Workshop course.

DRIVING THE MESSAGE HOME

When it comes to adherence to medication, remembering to take your meds is crucial. However, as you know, remembering does not always happen.

The human mind is complex, and so are our memories. Sometimes we remember correctly, and sometimes remember incorrectly.

The following TED Talk by Psychologist Elizabeth Loftus discusses the flip side of memory: false memory. She addresses when people either remember things that didn't happen or remember them differently from the way they really were.

This is crucial when it comes to adherence. How many times have we gotten to the end of the day and wondered if we had or had not taken our meds that day?

How often do we make it to the end of the week and think we adhered perfectly when we missed several doses?

Enjoy this discussion of false memories, and use it as an inspiration to set a reminder for yourself. This way what you believe happened and what actually happened will be the same.

Watch 'How Reliable is Your Memory?' presented by Elizabeth Loftus on YouTube.

Integrating medication regimens into daily routines can improve adherence

For medications to be effective, they must be taken in the correct dosage at the right time, as prescribed by healthcare providers. The World Health Organization estimates that half of patients take their medications incorrectly, costing the U.S. health care system and consumers about $300 billion each year. In a new article, University of Missouri researchers say medication non-adherence interventions should be based on a personal systems approach that focuses on integrating medication taking into daily routines and involving supportive people who encourage taking medications correctly.

Cynthia Russell, associate professor of nursing, and Todd Ruppar, assistant professor in the Sinclair School of Nursing, say educating patients about the dangers and potential costs of taking medications improperly is not enough to change their behavior. Rather, Russell and Ruppar recommend taking a personal systems approach that involves assessing individuals' daily routines, proposing ways to make medication regimens easier, tracking adherence and evaluating whether the individual took the medications correctly.

"Previously, the focus has been on the personal characteristics of the patient such as knowledge about how the medication works, motivation to take it, depression and other cognitive barriers," Russell said. "Instead, we need to give patients practical ways to adhere to their medication regimens, like putting pills next to the coffee maker as a reminder to take them each morning or using technology like cell phones or computers to set reminders to take medications."

Russell and Ruppar say there are high costs associated with non-adherence, including hospitalizations, surgeries and wasted medications. If people took their medications as prescribed, they would likely save money and prevent additional health problems.

"Patients often go back to their health care providers saying their health has not improved, so they assume that their medication isn't working," Ruppar said. "Prescribers usually start with one drug, then recommend a combination of medications. However, if patients took them correctly they likely wouldn't need the additional drugs."

The researchers are also studying how electronic medication adherence monitoring influences patients' behaviors. Patients are given pill caps embedded with computer chips that record how many times they take their medications each day. The caps also provide feedback over a period of time that allows patients and their health care providers to see how many doses were missed and whether the medications were taken during a prescribed window of time.

Michelle Matteson, a doctoral student in the Sinclair School of Nursing, contributed to the research. The article, Improving Medication Adherence: Moving from Intention and Motivation to a Personal Systems Approach, was published in Nursing Clinics of North America.

From ScienceDaily

6 Characteristics of a good medication reminder

Apps, phone alarms, calendars, buddies…with so many options out there, it can be hard to make a decision about what kind of medication reminder system to use. Here are some guiding principles to look out for.

1. It works with your nature, not against it.
2. It adds a smile to your life. A medical condition is serious enough – look for ways to lighten things up!
3. It is 100% reliable. Not 60 or 85 or even 99 – 100.

Add your own:

4. ____

5. ____

6. ____

Take some time brainstorming in your journal about your experience with your medication, and then share your story with the Buddy and Soul community! Tag us on Instagram and Twitter @Buddy_N_Soul, using the **#BuddynSoulMedSupport**. By sharing with us on social media, not only can you help others with their personal journeys, you can read about those facing similar challenges.

The medication adherence reminder that finally stuck!

Hitting snooze on a reminder was my go-to move for a long time…Until I found the reminder that finally stuck and helped me boost my adherence. Here's how I got myself to stop snoozing, and start adhering.

Take some time brainstorming in your journal about your experience with your medication, and then share your story with the Buddy and Soul community! Direct message us YOUR story @Buddy_N_Soul on Instagram and be anonymously featured for a chance to **win a Buddy&Soul three month free membership**. You can also tag us on Instagram and Twitter @Buddy_N_Soul, using the **#BuddynSoulMedSupport**. By sharing with us on social media, not only can you help others with their personal journeys, you can read about those facing similar challenges.

Who needs a reminder when I've got a brain?

Reminder systems are proven to up adherence levels, but what ever happened to the good old-fashioned noggin? What say we drop the externals and get back to basics, shall we?

For:

1. Down with technology—I'm not an anarchist, but I'm definitely feeling that the more I'm wired to my phone the less I experience real life.
2. Technology is not flawless. Your battery can run low, or your phone can break. Your brain on the other hand is always attached to your head…we hope…
3. If I use this as an opportunity to train my brain, I'll have a gift I can take with me for the rest of my life.

Add your own argument:

4. ____

Against:

1. No, technology is not perfect, but neither is my brain. I forget a lot. Did I mention that I forget a lot?
2. My brain gets way more overloaded than my trusty phone. I'd much rather use my phone for storage and leave my brain open for other things.
3. If my brain were capable of reminding me to take my meds 100% of the time, I wouldn't be here. Obviously, relying only on memory isn't quite cutting it.

Add your own argument:

4. ____

You brush your teeth, yes? Twice a day?

How come there's no reminder system required for that? Well, because it's a habit. You are used to it, have embedded it in your routine, and have set, clear times for it, like before going to bed and immediately upon waking up in the morning.

Nobody roots for you or gives you candy, but you know that you did the right thing.

If you can turn taking your meds into a bona fide part of your routine, you're on the right track.

Defining a time and method for taking your medication will help a lot, relieving you of the when-do-I-need-to-take-its and the darn-I-forgot-agains and, of course, the dreaded how-could-I-not-have-brought-the-meds!

Habits make life easier, put us on the right path, and regulate our lives.

The habit needs to consist of a trigger (e.g. *when I wake up, right before lunch,* or *at 7 pm*), an action (e.g. *taking my medication)* and a reward (e.g. watching my favorite show).

And here's the rub:

When you use an external reward, like a piece of chocolate or a bought cup of coffee (pending dietitian approval), you risk not complying with the action if the reward runs out. This is an acceptable risk to run if you're trying to get more leisure reading done in the evenings. If you fall a chapter behind in your novel because you don't have your chocolatey goodness on hand it's no big disaster. But when dealing with our medication, we should probably run a tighter ship.

The way to do that is to truly make it a habit, like brushing teeth or saying, "bless you" when someone sneezes.

And one of the best ways to make a new habit stick is to tack it onto an existing habit.

So let's do it.

Use your journal to **list what you'll use for your trigger, action, and reward for taking your meds.**

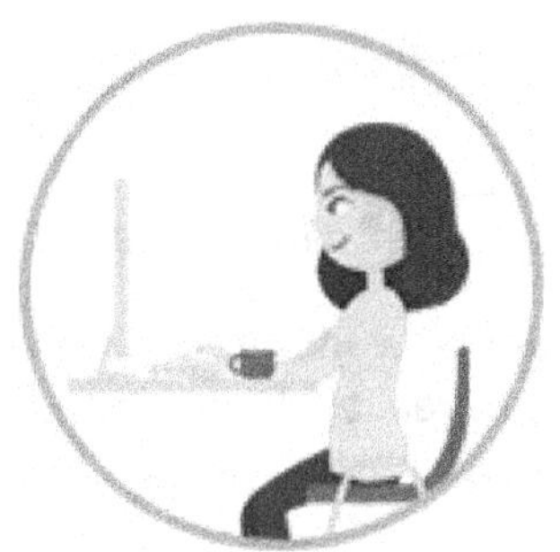

1. **Trigger.** This will be a current habit you have that can accommodate med-taking (e.g. brushing my teeth in the morning).
2. **Action.** This will be taking your meds.
3. **Reward.** Preferably something internal – like a sense of accomplishment – but a small treat works just fine too.

TIPS

Tip 1: Check out the Buddy&Soul Habit Workshop course for a more comprehensive guide to forming and sustaining habits.

Tip 2: To make the habit extra-effective, see what best supports you in taking your medication. For example – having a water bottle with you, the easier to swallow the pill; having a snack in your bag, in case you missed a meal but need to take your meds after eating, etc. If you include these in your routine, your adherence will improve.

Dan Pink, career analyst, challenges the very structure that most businesses are built on.

"If you want people to perform better, you reward them. Right?" He asks. "Bonuses, commissions, their own reality show. Incentivize them. That's how business works." And yet, the research shows the quite the opposite.

Pink says, "You've got an incentive designed to sharpen thinking and accelerate creativity, and it does just the opposite. It dulls thinking and blocks creativity."

So how can we best reward ourselves for taking our meds? By moving toward internal rewards, and away from external ones.

Watch 'The Puzzle of Motivation' presented by Dan Pink at TEDGlobal on www.ted.com

8 Internal motivators to help up your adherence

Intrinsic motivation is the way to go if you want to establish a lasting habit of adhering to your meds.
Here are some great intrinsic motivators to help you feel rewarded for taking your meds.

1. I am keeping my body healthy.
2. I have self-discipline and can take my medications when I need to.
3. Every pill is a step in the right direction.
4. I love my body and myself.
5. Every time I take my meds I'm reminding myself how much I love my family and am giving to them by staying healthy.

Add your own:

6. ____

7. ____

8. ____

Take some time brainstorming in your journal about your experience with your medication, and then share your story with the Buddy and Soul community! Tag us on Instagram and Twitter @Buddy_N_Soul, using the **#BuddynSoulMedSupport**. By sharing with us on social media, not only can you help others with their personal journeys, you can read about those facing similar challenges.

Should you use bribes to motivate you to take your meds?

They say that external rewards don't work, but for plenty of us, a scoop of ice cream offers more motivation than a "sense of accomplishment." As long as it works, does it really make a difference if your motivation is intrinsic or extrinsic?

For:

1. You have a medical condition *and* you're expected to adhere to your meds. Sheesh. No need to impose extra restrictions upon yourself.
2. If it works, go with it. Just make sure not to run out of your treat of choice anytime soon!

Add your own argument:

3. ____

Against:

1. It may work now, but it won't work in the long run.
2. A treat is so temporary. Why sell yourself short and miss the opportunity to create real, lasting behavioral change?
3. I always do what the doctors order. If they say intrinsic motivation, then that's what I'll go for.

Add your own argument:

4. ____

The trigger that finally made me take my meds

It took a few swings and misses, but you finally found the trigger that allowed you to take your meds, and to stick to taking your meds. It's no small feat — so share with the community how you finally found the right trigger.

Take some time brainstorming in your journal about your experience with your medication, and then share your story with the Buddy and Soul community! Tag us on Instagram and Twitter @Buddy_N_Soul, using the **#BuddynSoulMedSupport**. By sharing with us on social media, not only can you help others with their personal journeys, you can read about those facing similar challenges.

The reward that successfully got me to take my meds

How did you finally find the reward that got you to take your meds? What were some of the rewards that you tried and they simply didn't work? Share with the community, and help others who are facing similar challenges with reward-setting.

Direct message us YOUR story @Buddy_N_Soul on Instagram and be anonymously featured for a chance to **win a Buddy&Soul three month free membership**.

Strategy 10: Engage the power of your thoughts

According to *Motivational Interviewing* by William
Miller and Stephen Rollnick, research has found that a
patient's motivation to adhere to treatment is influenced
by his or her degree of confidence in being able to follow
it.

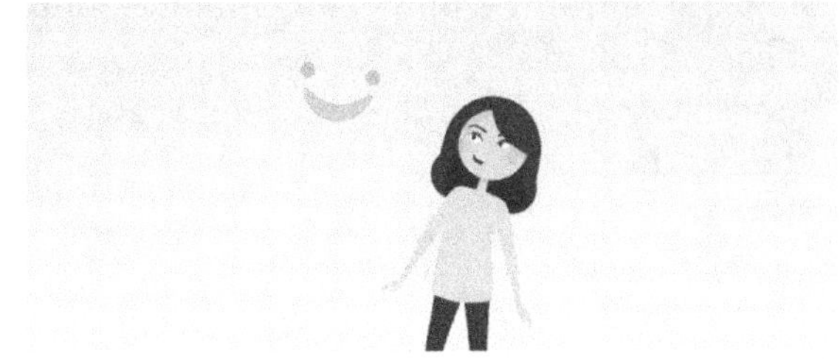

**In other words, you may believe in your treatment, but
if your following thought is, "there's no way I'll be able
to follow this treatment plan," you likely won't adhere
to it very well.**

Now that you've gotten all the knowledge about your medication, have explored alternatives, have set
up reminders, and have created a habit, it's time to put on the finishing touch to adherence by
harnessing your thoughts.

But how can you change your thoughts? Either you have confidence in your ability to adhere, or you
don't, right? Can anything be done to genuinely boost your confidence in your ability to do this and stick
with it?

According to author Brian Tracy in his book *The Power of Self-Confidence,* the answer is a resounding
yes! You do have the power to change your thoughts and your self-confidence in being able to
successfully follow your treatment plan. "Anything that you think about long enough and hard enough
eventually becomes a part of your mental processes, exerting its influence and power on your attitude
and your behavior" (p. 3).

Your thoughts influence your feelings, which influence your actions (remember, if you think global
warming is a sham, you probably won't conserve energy or recycle). The more you think about your
success in your treatment plan, the greater your self-confidence will be, and the more likely you'll be to
follow through.

Your positive thoughts have the power to link success to your treatment.

EXERCISE

Find or create an empowering mantra about sticking to your medication.
It can be something like, "I love my body and I will show it love by taking my medication" or, "Just like I succeed at showering every day, so too will I take these pills."

Write your mantra in your journal.

And congratulate yourself on reaching the end of the Adhering to Your Medication course!

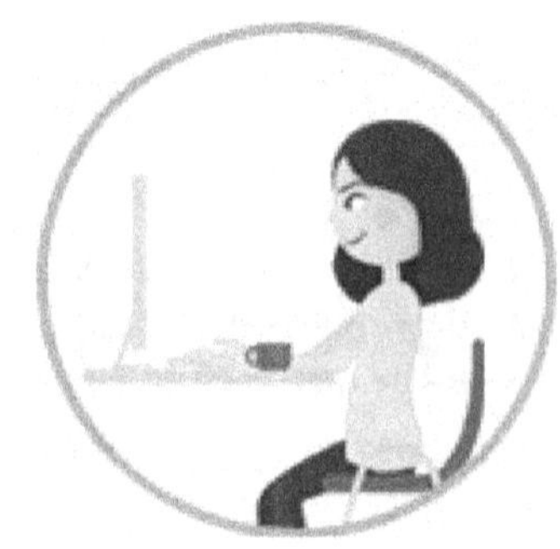

TIPS

Tip 1: There are no rules here – it's whatever feels right for you. The more airtime you give this positive thought, the more it will become part of your being, increasing your self-confidence, even if you don't 100% believe it at first.

Tip 2: Repeat your mantra at fixed times and situations, like while brushing your teeth.

Tip 3: Revisit your journal any time to modify, revise, or add to your mantra.

Tip 4: For more on making lasting change in your life, check out our Tackling Change course. 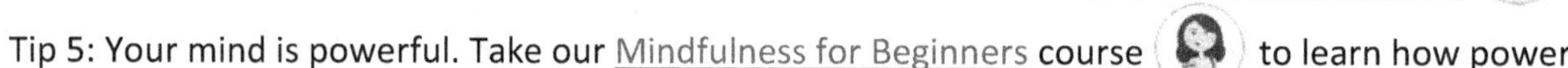

Tip 5: Your mind is powerful. Take our Mindfulness for Beginners course to learn how powerful.

Brian Tracy is Chairman and CEO of Brian Tracy International, a company specializing in the training and development of individuals and organizations.

He is an entrepreneur, public speaker, best-selling author and success expert. When it comes to self-confidence, he is an expert.

Watch Tracy describe the three main obstacles to self-confidence and how confidence, or lack of confidence, will influence your thoughts and behaviors.

If your confidence is low, your adherence is also probably low. So give yourself a confidence boost, and an adherence boost, and change directions from failure to success with your treatment plan.

Watch 'Become Self Confident' presented by Brian Tracy on YouTube.

Can a mantra help you improve your adherence?

There are all these techniques out there to help with medication compliance. Some of them seem promising, but a mantra? Seriously? That won't do squat.

For:

1. New Age things like mantras and chakras might work if you're New Age. But what about the rest of us?
2. I'm not much of an optimist. And I don't think a tell-it-as-it-is mantra is all that inspiring.
3. Nothing can help my adherence. It's just that bad.

Add your own argument:

4. ____

Against:

1. What do I have to lose? There's no harm in trying.
2. A mantra only takes a few seconds to say. A worthwhile effort if it could mean upping my medication adherence.
3. Positive mantras have proven effective in other areas. What's to say they won't be effective here?

Add your own argument:

4. ____

10 Things I learned about myself when I upped medication adherence

Sometimes challenging yourself to stick to something that you know will help you has far-reaching impacts on other areas of your life. In addition to adherence, what else has taking your meds taught you about yourself?

1. I learned I could stand up for myself and confidently talk to my medical team. I used to think people in white coats wouldn't listen to my concerns.
2. I learned to put on my big badge and swallow my bitter pill.
3. I learned I could maturely offer myself rewards without getting carried away.
4. I'm no longer scared of big words and science. This is about me and my body.
5. I've learned to advocate for myself without being shy or embarrassed.
6. I can put my negative feelings aside in order to do the right thing.
7. I've learned to take my intuition seriously. If something feels wrong, it might actually *be* wrong.

Add your own:

8. ____

9. ____

10. ____

The surprising connection I discovered between self-confidence and taking my meds

Share with the community how you built self-confidence, and how that impacted your adherence. You may be able to inspire others to do the same!

Take some time brainstorming in your journal about your experience with your medication, and then share your story with the Buddy and Soul community! Tag us on Instagram and Twitter @Buddy_N_Soul, using the **#BuddynSoulMedSupport**. You can also direct message us YOUR story @Buddy_N_Soul on Instagram and be anonymously featured for a chance to **win a Buddy&Soul three month free membership**. By sharing with us on social media, not only can you help others with their personal journeys, you can read about those facing similar challenges.

How low self-confidence was impacting my adherence

You may not have thought it was connected, but self-confidence can be a huge player in the field of adherence to medication. Share with the community how your self-confidence sabotaged your adherence to your medication.

You can also direct message us YOUR story @Buddy_N_Soul on Instagram and be anonymously featured for a chance to **win a Buddy&Soul three month free membership**.

7 Reasons not to take a 'medication vacation'

When you go on vacation, you might be tempted to leave your meds at home, along with the bills and the rain boots. But taking a 'medication vacation' is never a good idea. Here are a few reasons why.

1. Your body may be on vacation, but your health is not. A week of good times vs. your long-term health... Hm...
2. The last thing you want on vacation is to disrupt your health by not taking meds. You won't be able to enjoy yourself because you won't be feeling up to par.
3. It's hard enough to maintain your balance when you're in a different place and on a different schedule. Throw stopping with your meds into the mix and your body will just be downright disoriented.
4. Popular ideas don't equal smart ideas. A lot of people may do it, but what are the stats on how many of them emerge unscathed, so to speak?
5. Instead of thinking of your meds as something that restricts you, think of them as something that allows you to function, and to go on vacation!
6. Watch *Lorenzo's Oil* to see how intensely people worked to create a cure for an illness. Do you still want to take your medication so lightly?
7. Not taking your meds can bring up a lot of emotional turmoil, such as guilt, shame, embarrassment etc. Do you really want to bring that all up on vacation?

You've finished the Adhering to Your Medication book, but you haven't finished the journey. It doesn't end, it just gets better. Revisit this book, carry its ideas with you. Check out BuddynSoul.com and the rest of our books for all we have to offer. Spread the word. And change your life for good.

Create a Pleasant Reality.

Whether you've found yourself struggling with depression or are just looking to make your day-to-day life more enjoyable, this book is for you. We've created this book as a multimedia tool for you to learn how to create a pleasant reality. You can do it. And we all need it.

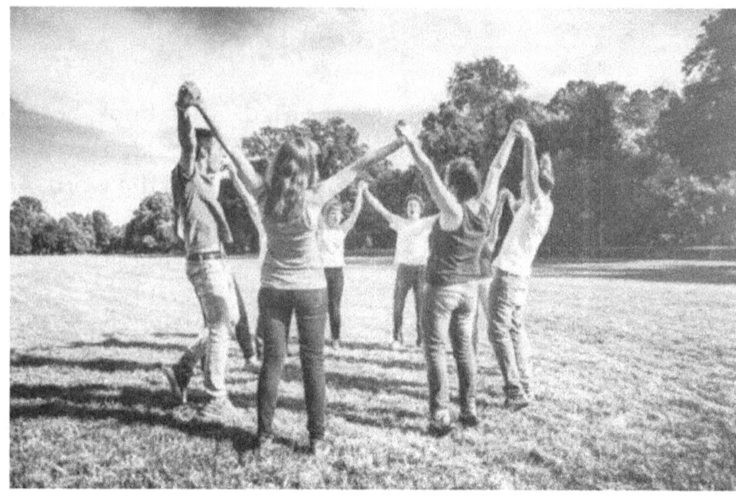

Goals you can achieve from reading 'Create a Pleasant Reality':

1. Understand what holds you back from enjoying life.
2. Learn tools to change the things you can and embrace the things you can't.
3. Tap into the power of ordinary moments to add joy and meaning to your life.

Manage your Medical Condition.

Being diagnosed with a medical condition is just the start. It marks the beginning of a journey into the unknown. And, whether you like it or not, on this journey, you are the captain of that boat! Or at least, the co-captain, alongside your physician. Because, let's face it, there are very few situations in which your involvement is not at all required. Even by opening your mouth to swallow a pill.

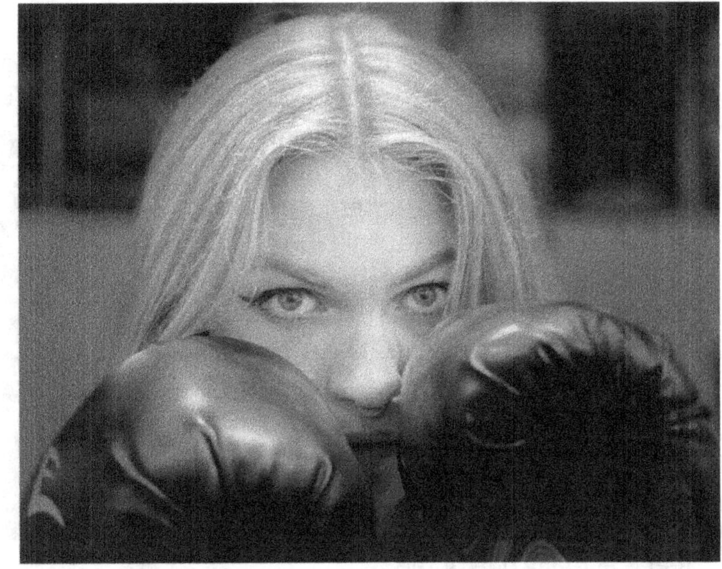

Goals you can achieve from reading 'Manage your Medical Condition':

1. Gain tools to actively manage your health.
2. Learn how to sort through and interpret medical information.
3. Assume responsibility for how you manage your medical condition.

Emotionally Managing your Illness.

Being ill is not easy. A lot is going on, and very little of it is fun. Being asked "how are you feeling?" might be nice the first few thousand times, but eventually it seems either redundant (I feel terrible! Still! But thanks for asking…) or like a sham (I'm falling apart at the seams, but I'll beam a smile and say "fine" because I don't have the energy to entertain pity). It may also seem beside the point, because you are ill, physically unwell, so what else is there to know? But, connecting with how you feel is actually one of the most important parts of having and managing a disease.

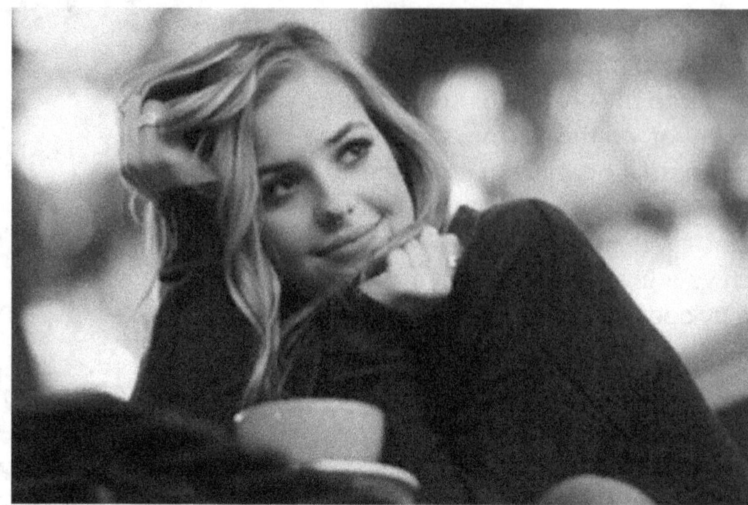

Goals you can achieve from reading 'Emotionally Managing Your Illness':

1. Identify, map out and sort your feelings regarding your illness.
2. Find strength and emotional balance to see you through your medical condition.
3. Take responsibility for your emotional well-being during your illness.

WANT TO LEARN MORE? CHECK THESE OUT!

MOVIES

Lorenzo's Oil (1992)

Based on a true story, this movie depicts the struggles of a father trying to find a cure for his son's rare, degenerative disease. The movie shows how far parents are willing to go to keep their child alive and how the medical world can justifiably be challenged and improved by laymen.

This movie is an inspiring reminder that sometimes, you have to be hands-on with your own treatment.

My Left Foot (1989)

The true story of Christy Brown, an Irishman paralyzed from birth by Cerebral Palsy. While his doctors deemed him to be retarded, his mother taught him to use the one part of his body he could control – his foot – to perform numerous activities. Brown was a successful writer, painter, and fundraiser despite his disability.

This movie will inspire people who are feeling discouraged by the limitations their medical conditions impose upon them.

APPS

MedSimple

This app not only reminds you to take your meds, but also provides information about alternate and generic medications you can purchase if yours is not in stock. It also stores a list of your doctors and pharmacies and reminds you when it's time to buy refills for your various medications.

This app is great for people who travel often and need to make sure they will always have enough meds with them until they return home.

NeedyMeds Alert

If being reminded when to take your medication isn't enough for you, this app will also give you in depth information about how your medication is treating your condition, how it may interact with other medications you take, and what side-effects you may experience while taking it.

A useful app for anyone who needs context and information in order to adhere to their medication.

BOOKS

How to Take Charge of Your Health: Handbook to Navigate Today's Medical Visits by Susan Cooper

This book gives you tips for making the most of your medical visits, as long as you are of sound enough mind and body to ask questions and make your wishes known. Advice about what to do and where to go in a medical emergency are an extra bonus.

Perfect for people who want to get the best bang for their buck, even in a doctor's office.

Patient Compliance with Medications: Issues and Opportunities by Jack E. Fincham

While this book was written for health professionals, people who have a chronic need for medication – as well as their relatives and caretakers – will benefit from what it has to offer. Topics covered include: the prevalence and cost of failing to take medications, the role of health care professionals in combating such noncompliance, and practical tips for dealing with this problematic phenomenon.

It is best to read this book *before* you start to get lax in taking your medications and nip non-adherence in the bud!

GADGETS AND PRODUCTS

Medcenter Talking Alarm Clock And Medication Reminder

This helpful talking alarm clock can remind you to take your medication up to 4 times daily. It features a friendly female voice that can be programmed with additional pleasant messages, such as good morning. It is battery operated, and small enough to carry around with you.

Perfect for those who need auditory reminders to adhere to their medication.

The e-pill Cadex 12 Alarm Medication Reminder Watch – Black

Are you someone who's constantly on the move? So why not take your adherence-reminders with you...right on your wrist! This medication-reminder watch can hold up to 12 different alarms per day with both sound and/or text reminders. It has a snooze option to give you periodical reminders every 3 minutes until you take your pills. It also offers a medical alert databank, which displays your medical information in case of an emergency.

This gadget can take care of the technical side of adhering to your medication.